Winnie & Her Worries

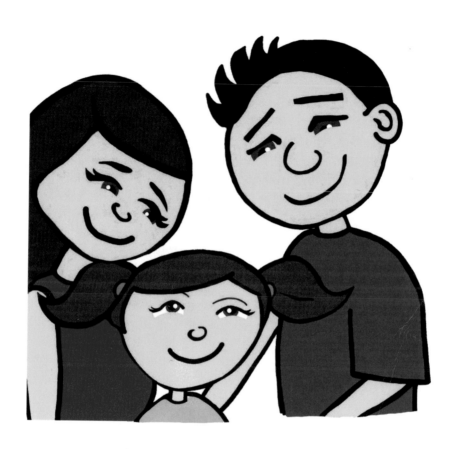

By Reena B. Patel, MA, LEP, BCBA

Illustrated by Jared Hogue

Edited by Avanti Pradhan Vadivelu
KIND EYE PUBLISHING, LLC

To anyone who struggles with stress and anxiety - You are never alone and we CAN change the ending!

To my husband Bijal for being my biggest fan.

To my children - Ayana, Maliya, and Jivaan. My wish for you is to grow up with the confidence to BE YOU. Nothing will ever be so powerful.

To my nieces and nephew - Nalini, Ashni, Sahana, Mila and Dhillon. I love you always!

To Chev - Thank you for your tremendous help with the final stages of this book.

My name is Winnie and I love waking up on Sunday mornings and making pancakes with my dad. We love to flip them up in the air and try catching them on our plates.

I also love spending my afternoons playing catch at the park with my dog, Sir London.

And I love to spend the evenings reading stories with my mom while I sit with her on our rocking chair.

I feel happy and warm inside when I have these thoughts inside my head.

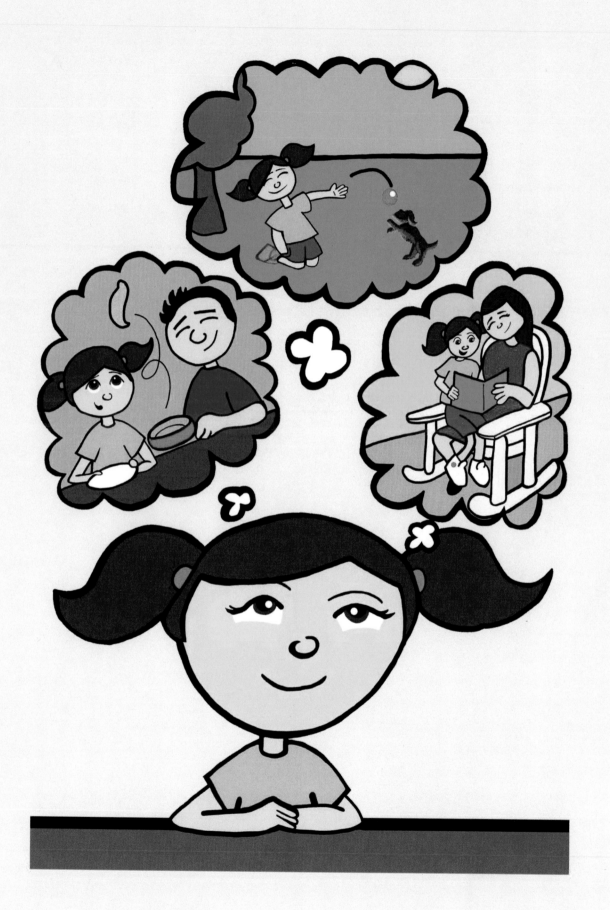

But sometimes, I have thoughts that make me feel worried instead of happy.

What if I don't make it to the bus on time?

What if I don't finish my homework tonight?

Will my friend Maliya sit next to me at lunch tomorrow?

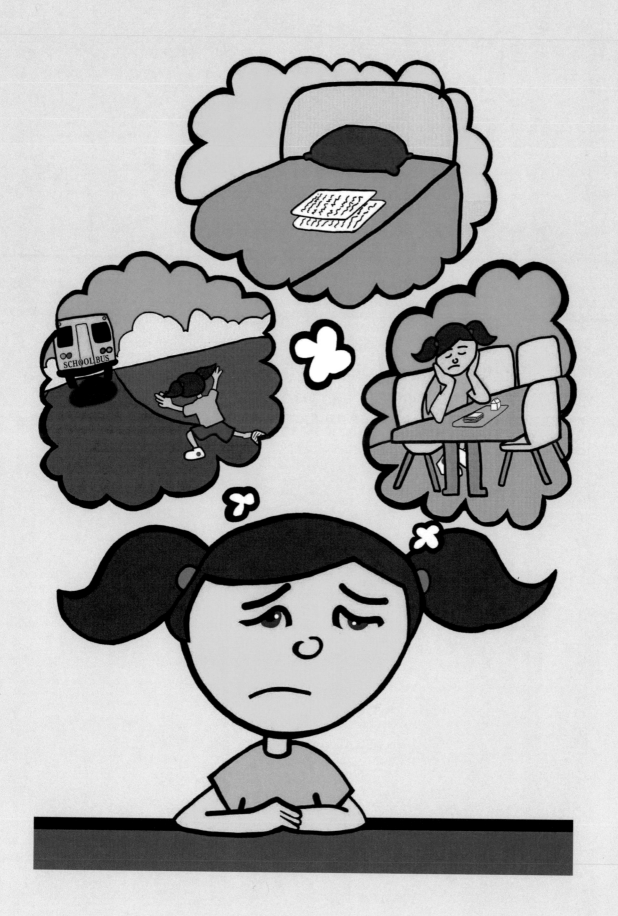

When I feel worried, my brain feels like something wrong or stressful is about to happen. It goes into protective mode and prepares my body to defend itself.

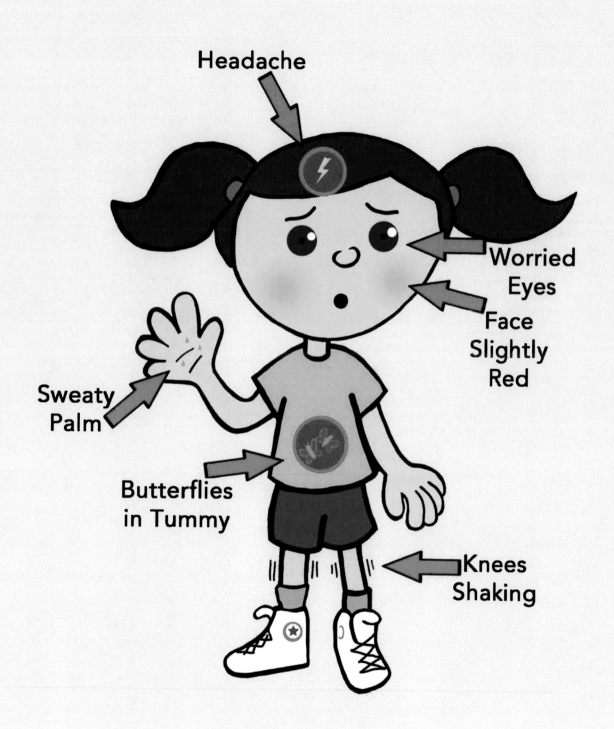

Sometimes these worries build up when I am at school and I start to panic and begin to cry. When this happens I just want to go home and hide under the covers in my bed.

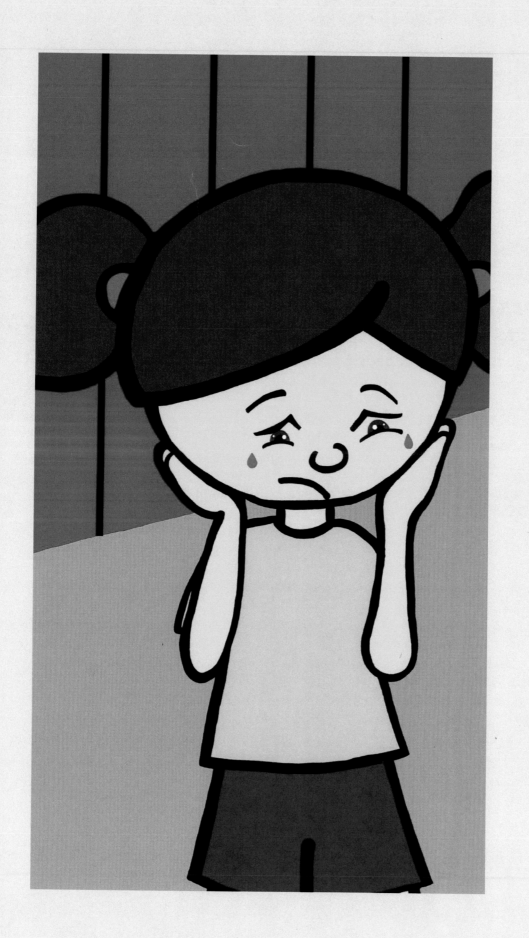

I know my parents are always there to help when I start to feel this way. They say that feeling worried is common and happens to everyone, even grown-ups. We can feel worried before a test, when meeting new people, or wondering who to sit next to at lunch.

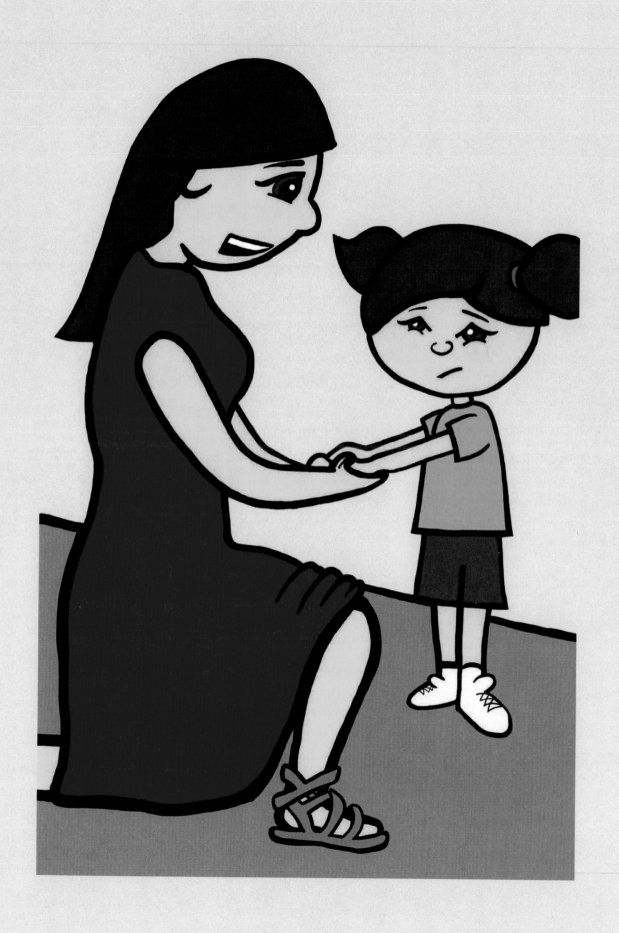

But, we can be in charge of those worry thoughts, and there are ways we can turn them into happy thoughts. This is great, because I feel sad when my worries get in the way of doing the activities I love, like going to school and playing with my friends.

When I feel worried, my parents remind me of the different ways, or *coping strategies*, I can use to fight the worries.

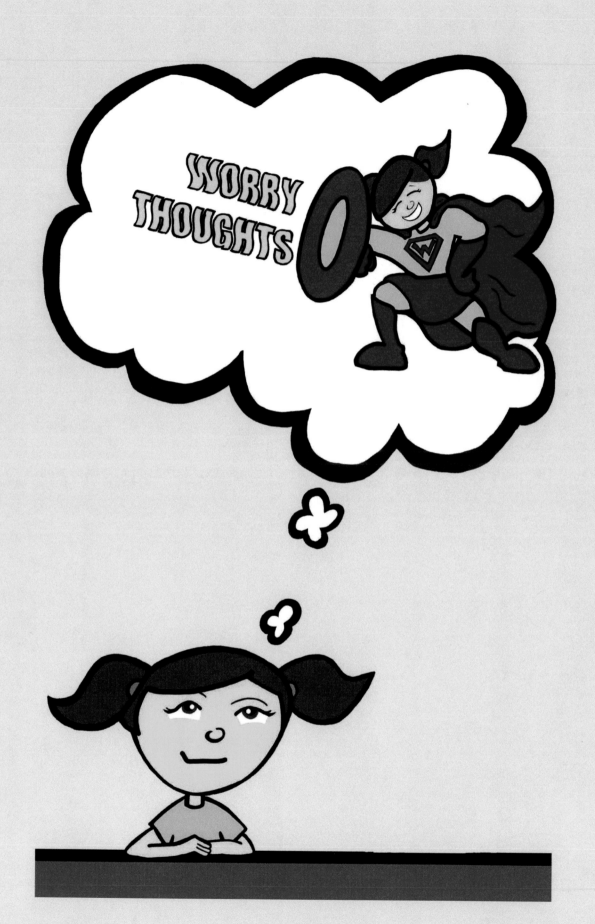

But first, it's important to recognize that my thoughts are worries and those feelings are real, which is OK! This is called *Self-Awareness*. My parents taught me this.

Next, we act like detectives and identify what is making me feel worried, and how it's affecting my body and brain.

Mom & Dad remind me that it's OK to talk about my worries out loud. My parents even share worries that they had when they were my age. This makes me feel more at ease.

My parents always remind me that they are there to support me and that I am safe. If I'm at school, my teacher does the same thing. I feel very loved.

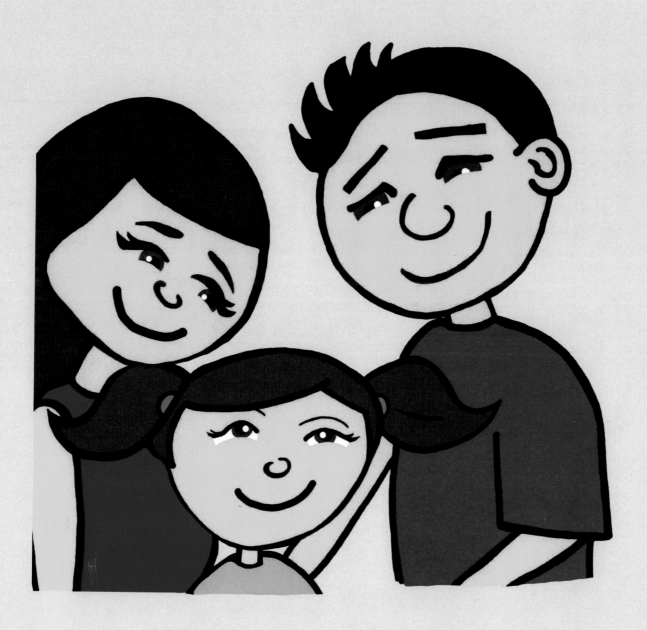

One of my favorite coping strategies I learned to use is called the *"worry box"* . This is when I write down my worry thoughts on small strips of paper and drop it into a box. I even decorated my box with stickers! Once my worries are in there I don't have to keep thinking about them because they are contained in the box.

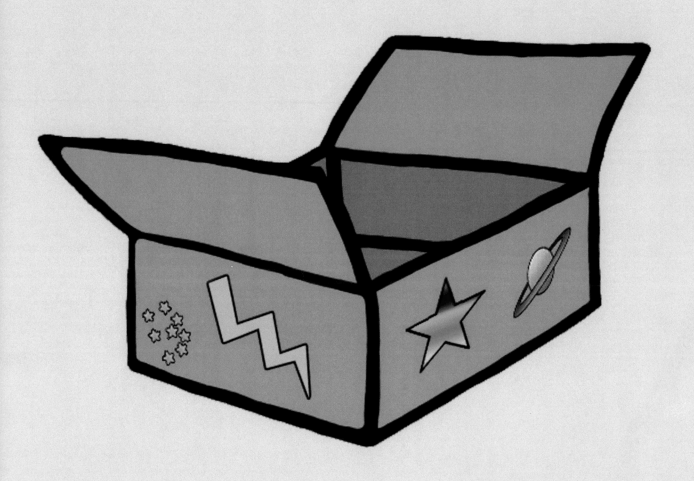

My parents and I then pick a time of day to read through the worries together. We call that "W Time" and we talk about any worries I had throughout the day and how I can work through them.

The next morning I woke up and got ready for school. As I was walking into class a worry thought popped into my head, "what if I forget to bring my book home today?" This time, all by myself, I remembered the tools my parents and I came up with. I felt in charge of my thoughts and I was able to stop my worries!

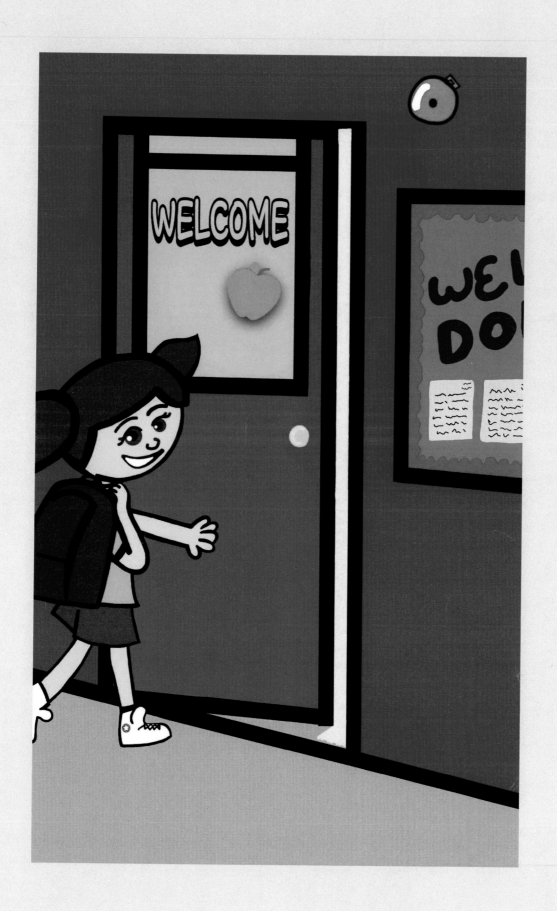

TOOLS for Parents and Educators

It is important for children to learn to manage their emotions and feelings when faced with stressors, or "triggers", by helping them develop coping strategies.

When implementing any of the strategies suggested below, the single most important first step is to create a safe and loving judgment free space built on trust. The next step is to remember that children are all different and what works well for one child might not work well for another. Finally, it is important to learn that managing symptoms of stress and anxiety takes time and practice.

Coping Strategies

COME BACK

When the child catches themselves being caught up in worries about the future or guilt and regret about the past, help them notice what is happening and simply and kindly remind them to say to themselves, "come back." Then, remind them to take a calming breath and focus on what they are doing in the moment.

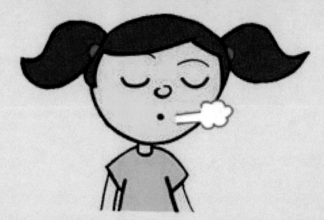

THREE SENSES

Help the child become aware of what they are experiencing in the moment through their three senses - sound, sight, and touch. Ask them to take a few slow breaths while asking themselves:

- What are three things I can hear?

- What are three things I can see?

- What are three things I can feel?

Ask the child to think of these answers to themselves slowly, one sense at a time.

BODY SCAN

The aim of this exercise is to bring awareness to the physical sensations in different parts of the child's body. Their minds are probably used to labeling these sensations as good or bad, uncomfortable, or even painful. See if you can help them notice what they feel without judging themselves.

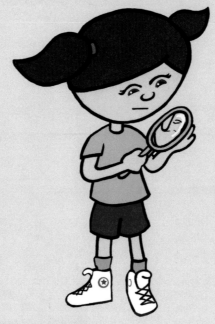

MINDFUL BREATHING WITH FINGERS

Children can use their hand as a visual model to help them concentrate on their breathing. Becoming more aware and providing sensory input through the gentle sensations can be calming as well. Children concentrate on taking five slow breaths in through their nose and out through their mouths. Children may need to practice this first, as they may be mouth breathing. If you notice that your child finds breathing through their nose a challenge, invite them to imagine that they are smelling a beautiful flower or their favorite food as they breathe in, and then to breathe out with a big sigh. (Breathing in and smelling a beautiful smell and breathing out with a sigh because it smelled so good.) At the same time as breathing, children will focus on the action of tracing up and down the fingers of one hand and the gentle sensations this creates.

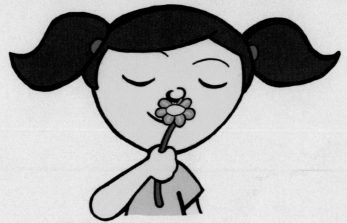

WORRY BOX

A great activity for children struggling with worries and anxiety is creating a "worry box". This activity can be as simple or as elaborate as you would like. Children decorate a box however they like, such as with glitter, markers, stickers, etc. As they are crafting their box, explain that the box will be a spot in which they keep their worries when they don't have the time to think about them. They write their worry on a piece of paper and place it in a box to be addressed at a later time. It gives children a sense of control over their worries, and parents can set aside a certain time of day to talk to children about their fears. When they no longer feel as though they need to address a certain worry that is in the box, the piece of paper can be ripped up and thrown in the garbage, which can be therapeutic as well.

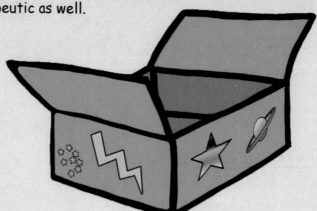

POSITIVE MANTRA BRACELET

Making positive mantra bracelets is a simple but fun way to get children talking about positive thinking and, more specifically, which mantras best apply to them and their worries. Start by opening up a discussion about the things they worry about most, and help them come up with three or four mantras they can repeat to themselves in an worry moment, such as "I am safe", "Mom will always come back," or "My best is good enough". Assign each mantra to a different bead, and have them string them onto a pipe cleaner or lanyard to be worn on their wrist as a daily reminder to think positive thoughts and breathe. The soft pipe cleaner and smooth, sliding beads also function as an awesome yet discreet fidget for our tactile seeking little ones.

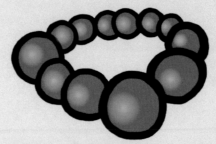

For more information regarding coping strategies for children with worries, please visit www.autizmandmore.com

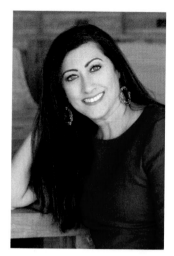

Reena Patel, MA, LEP, BCBA, has had the privilege of working with families and children supporting all aspects of education and positive wellness for the past two decades as a Guidance Counselor, Licensed Educational Psychologist, and Board Certified Behavior Analyst. Ms. Patel has worked extensively with typically developing children as well as with children with exceptional needs, supporting their academic, behavioral and social and emotional development. She has found with the expectations and challenges our children currently face, it is imperative to teach children the proper tools to address stress and anxiety.

Reena routinely holds workshops throughout California, guiding and training parents and educators on practical techniques that are easy to implement. Ms. Patel lives in San Diego, California with her husband and three children. She would like to remind us all to "be grateful, be present, be you".

For more information regarding the author and her practice, **AutiZm & More**, **please visit www.autizmandmore.com.**

Kind Eye Publishing, LLC is a family owned & operated publishing company that promotes written pieces of work dedicated to the themes of kindness, compassion, inclusion and cross cultural communication. Our dream is to spread understanding through our published material, be it through magazines, essays, manuscripts, self-help books, how-to books and more. Our authors represent a diverse ethnic population and voices that may otherwise be unheard.

We invite you to speak your mind.

Someone is listening.

www.kindeyepublishing.com

Notes

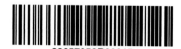

Made in the USA
San Bernardino, CA
13 June 2019